The Easy Keto Bread Cookbook 2021

Thomas Slow

Table of Contents

Introduction

Congratulations on purchasing *Keto Bread* and thank you for doing so. Inspiration for a special way of eating is what sent me on the keto journey. I have heard many good things about the plan as you too will soon discover. If you're new to the keto diet plan, let's discover a bit of the history of how the diet has traveled through time.

During the Paleogenic period, humans were known to hunt for their protein and gather their vegetables, fruits, nuts, and seeds to survive. Because this method isn't ideal in today's society; you don't have to search for food each day. That was the way people lived centuries ago which made the body develop a mechanism to survive during times when food was scarce.

Whenever a person encountered satiation where they consumed more calories than they burned, the unused calories would be converted into fat fuels and stored for emergency starvation times. This mechanism was useful in times where nutrient

4

resources were scarce and required a lot more energy to locate.

However, in modern times, food is not the only natural to come by, but most meals that are affordable are packed full of unnecessary calories. Your body will continue to create these fat stores, even though the times of hunting and gathering are behind us. These facts were taken into consideration when the ketogenic diet was developed.

The only way to lose fat is to trick the body into burning it. If you specifically consume meals high in fats and very low-lacking in carbohydrates; your body will believe that the only fuel available is fat. It will then enter what is known as ketosis; the process whereby the liver releases more ketones. Thus, ketones form as a result of burning fats for fuels.

Starvation mode is known when the body is calorie deficient and lacking in the nutrients it needs. Many people have forced his/her bodies into starvation mode in a desperate attempt to lose weight. However, what few people realize is that the weight loss while in starvation mode is usually muscle tissue. The body holds onto its emergency fat stores until the last possible moment. A ketosis is a form of starvation mode that takes this fat away. You won't be depriving your body of calories or nutrients. You will be starving your body of carbohydrates and sugars.

During the era of the 1920s and 1930s, the ketogenic diet was prevalent for its role in epilepsy therapy treatments. The diet plan provided another method other than the uncharacteristic techniques of fasting which were victorious in the treatment plan. During the 1940s, the process was abandoned because of new therapies for seizures. However, approximately 20 to 30% of the epileptic cases failed to reach control of epileptic seizures. With that failure, the keto diet was reintroduced as a management technique.

The Charlie Foundation was founded by the family of Charlie Abraham in 1994 after his recovery from seizures and other health issues he suffered daily. Charlie—as a youngster—was placed on the diet and continued to use it for five years. As of 2016, he is still functioning successfully without the seizure episodes and is furthering his education as a college student.

The Charlie Foundation appointed a panel of dietitians and neurologists to form an agreement in the form of a statement in 2006. It was written as an approval of the diet and stated which cases its use would be considered. It is noted that the plan is especially recommended for children. The plan continues to improve as time passes and more research is completed.

Chapter 1: Overview Of A Ketogenic Diet

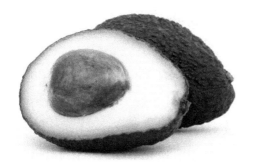

Why Keto Is So Effective For Weight Loss?

If you don't consume enough carbs from your food, your cells will begin to burn fat for the necessary energy instead. Your body will switch over to ketosis for its energy source as you cut back on carbs and calories.

Two elements that occur when your body doesn't need the glucose:

- *The Stage of Lipogenesis:* If there is a sufficient supply of glycogen in your liver and muscles, any excess is converted to fat and stored.

- *The Stage of Glycogenesis*: The excess of glucose converts to glycogen and is stored in the muscles and liver. Research indicates that only about half of your energy used daily can be saved as glycogen.

Your body will have no more food (similar to when you are sleeping) making your body burn the fat to create ketones. Once the ketones break down the fats, which generate fatty acids, they will burn-off in the liver through beta-oxidation. Thus, when you no longer have a supply of glycogen or glucose, ketosis begins and will use the consumed/stored fat as energy.

Principles of the Keto Diet

The keto diet will set up your body to deplete the stored glucose. Once that is accomplished, your body will focus on diminishing the stored fat you have saved as fuel. Many people don't understand that counting calories don't matter at this point since it is just used as a baseline. Your body doesn't need glucose which will trigger these two stages:

The State of Glycogenesis: The excess of glucose converts itself into glycogen which is stored in the muscles and liver. Research indicates only about <u>half</u> of your energy used daily can be saved as glycogen.

The State of Lipogenesis: This phase is introduced when there is an adequate supply of glycogen in your liver and muscles, with any excess being converted to fat and stored.

Your body will have no more food (similar to the times when you are sleeping) making your body burn the fat to create ketones. Once the ketones break down the fats, which generate fatty acids, they will burn-off in the liver through beta-oxidation. Thus, when you no longer have a supply of glycogen or glucose, ketosis begins and will use the consumed/stored fat as energy.

When the glycerol and fatty acid molecules are released, the ketogenesis process begins, and acetoacetate is produced. The acetoacetate is converted to two types of ketone units:

Acetone: This is mostly excreted as waste but can also be metabolized into glucose. This is the reason individuals on a ketogenic diet will experience a distinctive smelly breath.

Beta-hydroxybutyrate or BHB: Your muscles will convert the acetoacetate into BHB which will fuel your brain after you have been on the keto diet for a short time.

How To Do It Right

You must decide how you want to proceed with your diet plan. It is always best to discuss this essential step with your physician. There are four methods, so you better understand the different levels of the keto diet plan. As a guideline, use these standards to stay within your chosen carbohydrate limits on the keto plan:

Method # 1: The standard ketogenic diet (SKD) is composed of moderate protein, high-fat, and is low in carbohydrates. Typically, this phase of the diet is considered a high-fat (75%), low-carbohydrate (5%), and moderate protein (20%) diet plan. These are average counts and can vary.

Method # 2: If you work out or are very active, you will call for the targeted keto diet which is also called TKD. The process involves adding additional carbohydrates to the diet plan during the times when you're more active.

Method # 3: The cyclical ketogenic diet (CKD) requires a restricted five-day keto diet plan followed by two high-carbohydrate days.

Method 4: The high-protein keto diet is comparable to the standard keto plan (SKD) in all aspects. You will consume more protein. Its ratio is repeatedly noted as maintaining 35% protein, 5% carbs, and 60% fat. (Once again, these are average percentages.)

The Internet provides you with several ways to calculate your daily intake of carbs. Try an easy to follow keto calculator for assistance. Begin your weight loss process by making a habit of checking your levels when you want to know what essentials your body needs during the course of your dieting plan. You will document your personal information such as height and weight. The Internet calculator will provide you with essential math.

Supplementation

The ketogenic diet has many benefits, but it's possible some of the essential nutrients are being overlooked in your menu planning. You may need to supplement to replace minerals including magnesium, potassium, calcium, and sodium which comes from some of the food items not used on the keto diet. These electrolytes control muscle and nerve function and many other issues. Below are just a few of the ways you can supplement your plan:

Add Fish Oil to your Diet: Purchase this at any health food store in either the liquid or capsule form. The oil provides a natural anti-inflammatory content and also contributes to the higher fat intake requirements on the ketogenic diet.

Use MCT Oils: Your ketogenic experience can improve with the use of MCT oil or medium-chain triglycerides. These fatty acids are found in its natural form in palm and coconut oil. Its advantages include the following:

- The oil helps lower your blood sugar.

- The use of MCTs makes it much easier to get into – and remain in ketosis. It is a natural anti-convulsive.

- It is also excellent for appetite control and weight loss.

Replace The Electrolytes: If you have a low level of electrolytes, especially potassium and sodium, you can frequently suffer from fatigue, headaches, and constipation which is commonly called keto flu. The low-carbs can also cause the kidneys to dump excess water, sodium, and other valuable electrolytes that must be replenished.

Consume Plenty of Sodium: The amount of sodium required differs from other diet plans because other plans generally focus on less sodium. The sodium is lost with the water loss, so you will need to increase the sodium intake to keep the right balance of electrolytes. This is crucial especially during the initial phase of the diet. Gain sodium in these ways:

- Drinking bone broth regularly

- Adding salt to your food - Himalayan sea salt is a good choice.

- Enjoy more sodium-rich foods including eggs and red meats

- Be sure to monitor your blood pressure because sodium can have an effect on your pressure levels if you're are prone to hypertension.

Increase Magnesium Intake: One of the most evident signs of a deficiency in magnesium is muscle cramps and fatigue. A blood test is the best way to test for possible problems. Magnesium has many benefits including proper nerve and muscle function, helps maintain normal heart rhythm, assists over 300 body reactions including supporting adequate testosterone levels and working with calcium to keep your bones healthy.

Ideally, men should consume 420 mg. daily; women need only 320 mg. Eat some of these foods to maintain adequate magnesium levels:

- Leafy green vegetables
- Pumpkin seeds
- Avocados
- Almonds
- High-fat yogurts

Consume More Potassium: Your normal blood pressure, regular heart rate, and fluid balance are aided by potassium. You need to remain cautious about adding potassium supplements to your diet because too much can cause an overload which could be toxic. Eat the following foods instead:

- Salmon
- Mushrooms
- Avocados
- Leafy greens
- Nuts

Chapter 2: Baking Basics

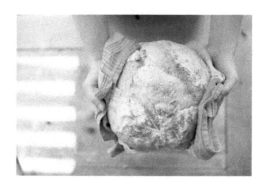

Equipment Needed

Baking Pans & Accessories:

Silicone Baking Mat: Make cleanup time simpler and keep your pans from slipping.

Ramekins: You will use these for melting butter and other various functions.

Square Baking Pans: You should check your recipes for specific sizes before baking. If you choose a smaller pan, it will take a bit longer to cook because it's deeper. The measurements should be a minimum of 2-inches deep. The sizes run from 8 to 9-inches.

Sheet Cake Pans: Use a 9x13-inch pan for breadsticks and many other bread options. Purchase a rimmed baking pan for any items that can easily slide off of the edges during preparation.

Muffin Pans: Muffin tins come in three popular sizes including mini, standard, and jumbo. The standard-size offers a .5 cup capacity with either 6 or 12 count cups. Mini tins provide one- cup capacity in both the 12 or 24-count cups and jumbo ones also provide one-cup capacity with a six-count tray. These are great for cupcakes and muffins. It's best to have a set of two so you can make larger batches without wasted time and money.

Pizza Pans or Pizza Stones: Purchase an array of sizes if you're a pizza lover. You can also use them for baking other goods also.

Wire Cooling Rack: The rack helps bread cool down quickly. Eliminate the steam that will build up in the baking pan which can make the bread loaves soggy on the bottom if cooled on a flat surface.

Other Essential Tools

- *Measuring Cups*: You should purchase sturdy measuring cups for dry ingredients. The oval types are much easier to reach into boxes for measurement.

- *Glass Measuring Cup*: Two and four cup measurement cups can also be used for mixing the ingredients. It also provides you a clear image of the contents to ensure proper measurement; no more eyeballing for accuracy.

- *Measuring Cups & Spoons*: Purchase a measuring cup and spoon system that shows both the Metric and US standards of weight so there is no confusion during prep. For dry ingredients, it's important to level off the product using a butter knife. When measuring liquids, be sure you have the measuring cup placed on a flat surface.

- *Measuring Spoons*: If possible, purchase spoons that have a magnet system, making storage much simpler. Never hunt for a spoon again!

- *Mixing Bowls*: Be sure to include a sturdy, four-quart capacity bowl which is excellent for most baking needs. Choose a clear container where you can see the contents of the breading process. However, keep two or three others to prevent interruptions after you begin the dessert preparations.

- *Flour Sifter:* Purchase a good sifter for under $10, and you will be ensured a more accurate measurement for your baking needs.

- *Rolling Pin*: Roll out your pastry shells easily using a rolling pin. Be creative if you do not have one to roll out your prepared dough.

- *Pastry Brush*: Consider using a silicone brush since the bristles won't stick together. Never stress over the leftover 'gunk' on the brush again! You can easily apply thin glazes or egg washes to ensure an even application.

- *Pastry Cutter:* Take minutes off of your preparation time using a cutter to blend in the butter to prepare the dough. Keep your hands clean!

- *Plastic Wrap/Kitchen Towel*: You should always have a clean kitchen towel handy for wiping your hands. You should have another towel set aside for covering your yeast bread products. If using plastic wrap, be sure to spray the side of the wrap facing the dough.

- *Nonstick Cooking Spray*: You can save cleanup time and much aggravation by preventing your baked goods from adhering to the baking pan.

- *Parchment Baking Paper & Aluminum Foil*: You can save tons of time by covering your baking pans and other cooking pots. The baking pans are lined with the paper/foil and the baked goods don't stick. For most baking needs, you can omit the oils if you choose the paper instead.

- *Dough Hook*: If you handle a lot of dough; make an investment of a dough hook to knead the dough with stationary or hand-held mixers right in the bowl.

- *Timer:* Many of your baking items are time-sensitive. Therefore, it's essential to properly time the rising of your dough items. Never burn a delicious loaf of bread again because the time passed you by!

Baking Skills Needed

Stages of bread baking are in existence when you prepare to bake and carry out the entire process of bread baking.

Mix The Raw Ingredients: In the case of bread, most of your raw ingredients consist mainly of water, yeast, salt, and flour. Then, you just combine them into the dough.

Sift the Flour – Or Not: If you take a page out of Grandma's book and sift the flour, it will aerate and remove any lumps from unsifted flour. The sifted flour is much lighter and is enriched with oxygen - making it easier to mix with other fixings - as you prepare the dough. After the flour is sifted, it is more likely to have an accurate measurement. When possible, always sift the flour.

Proof & Shape the Bread: The proofing phase of baking is where the yeast eats the sugar out of the flour. The result is that it and burps out gas and alcohol. As a result, the bread will rise to provide a natural - sweet flavor.

Baking the Bread: Baking is considered the stage where you apply the hot oven to your masterpiece. You will be creating a tasty and delicious treat. The final phase is the easiest, just enjoy the bread.

How Much To Knead:

Knowing how much to knead the bread product is just as essential as correct measurements of the items used in the recipe. You need to understand the ways to know when your bread is ready to bake. These are just a few of the hints of an excellent product every time:

The Dough Holds Its Shape: Once the kneading is successful, you can hold the bread in the air, and it will maintain its form. The ball shape means the gluten is 'strong' and tight.

The Dough Is Smooth: You will start noticing a lumpy – shaggy mass forming as you knead. The mixture should be just slightly tacky when touched.

Perform A Windowpane Test: Pull a portion of dough (tennis-ball size). Stretch it paper-thin. If it holds together, it's ready to bake. The 'true' point of kneading the dough is to strengthen the gluten (the stringy protein bands that provide texture to the bread. As a rule-of-thumb, it should take eight to ten minutes using a mixer or ten to twelve minutes if working the dough by hand.

Perform the Poke Test: Go ahead, and poke the mixture. If the hole fills in quickly, it's ready.

How To Know When Bread Is Done:

- *Visually Gauge Its Doneness:* With experience, you will learn how the bread's appearance changes during the cooking cycle. The color should be a deep golden brown and firm. Don't worry about the darker spots here-and-there; it's normal for home-baked bread.

- *Gently Tap The Bottom Of The Baking Pan:* This is a simple process. You take the pan out of the oven and turn it upside down on a flat surface. Tap the bottom, and it should sound hollow when the bread is done. Towards the end of the baking cycle, you can try this method every 5 minutes.

- *Check The Bread Internal Temperature:* Gently insert the thermometer into the center of the loaf of bread. Most bread is baked at $190°$ Fahrenheit. Once you add eggs, butter, or milk, the temperature averages $200°$ Fahrenheit.

What Dry Ingredients Can Be Used?

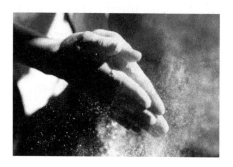

Flour Substitutes:

Almond Flour: Almond flour is considered an all-purpose flour and only contains 3 grams of carbs for .25 of a cup. You can prepare a batch by blanching the almonds in a pot of boiling water. Remove the skins. Grind the almonds into a fine flour to use for baking low-carb cookies, cakes, and pie crusts.

Coconut Flour: In addition to being high in fiber, coconut flour is high in protein. The same brand of coconut flour provides 19.3 grams of protein for every 100 grams. Like fiber, protein helps you stay full longer. It displays that tropical taste. Be sure it's stored in a closed container. Choose a spot where it's dark such as the pantry. The refrigerator and freezer could cause moisture contamination.

Almond Meal: Almond meal isn't the same as almond flour. It is a good substitute if you are out of almond flour for your baked goods. Merely throw a portion of almonds in a food processor to make the meal.

Flax Meal: Freshly milled meal preserves the natural nutrients and oil that flaxseed offers. You are provided with a health-giving digestive aid with its nutty taste. It also maintains natural cholesterol controllers with its high fiber content. Bake the delicious fiber into your recipes at 13 grams for just two tablespoons. Keep it refrigerated for freshness. You will receive about 4.25 cups per pound of the meal.

Sunflower Seed Or Pumpkin Seed Meal: You can receive high counts of vitamins and minerals including copper, vitamin E, phosphorus, thiamine, and selenium. You only gain 5 net carbs for every one-ounce serving. Use the same amount of sunflower seed meal or pumpkin seed meal as you do with almond meal flour since they have very similar properties.

Ground Psyllium Husk Powder: You will find this in several recipes. It is a binding agent with tons of fiber. This has fiber as its main ingredient but it is combined with other low-carb flours.

Whole Psyllium Husk: Use the entire husk in doughs where you require more 'stretchiness' such as what you would have in wheat flour. It's excellent for pizza dough, tortillas, or bread.

Sesame Flour: Finely grind sesame seeds to prepare the flour into a texture similar to wheat flour. Combine with psyllium flour for your baking needs to ensure the light texture of high-carb white bread.

Low-Carb Sweeteners Guide:

Erythritol Powder: The Purist is provided by NOW Foods has a 100% erythritol sweetener. The product is about 70% as sweet as sugar. Therefore, you need a little more. Start by using 1.33 to 1.5 teaspoons of the erythritol in comparison to one teaspoon of sugar.

Pyure Granulated Stevia: The best all-around sweetener is Pyure Organic All-Purpose Blend with less of a bitter aftertaste versus a stevia-based product. The blend of stevia and erythritol is an excellent alternative to baking, sweetening desserts, and various cooking needs.

The substitution ratio is one teaspoon of sugar for each one-third teaspoon of Pyure. Add slowly and adjust to your taste since you can always add a bit more. If you need powdered sugar, just grind the sweetener in a high-speed blender such as a NutriBullet until it's very dry.

Swerve Granular Sweetener: Swerve Granular Sweetener is also an excellent choice as a blend. It's made from non-digestible carbs sourced from starchy root veggies and select fruits. Start with 3/4 of a teaspoon for every one of sugar. Increase the portion to your taste. On the downside, it is more expensive (about twice the price) than other products such as the Pyure. You have to decide if it's worth the difference.

Swerve Confectioners Powdered Sugar for your baking needs. Unfortunately, it's more expensive (about twice the price) than other products such as the Pyure.

Xylitol (Granulated): Xylitol is at the top of the sugary list. It tastes just like sugar! The natural occurring sugar alcohol has the Glycemic index (GI) standing of 13. If you have tried others and weren't satisfied, this might be for you. Xylitol is also known to keep mouth bacteria in check which goes a long way to protect your dental health. The ingredient is commonly found in chewing gum. Unfortunately, if used in large amounts, it can cause diarrhea - making chewing gum a laxative if used in large quantities. *Pet Warning*: If you have a puppy in the house, be sure to use caution since it is toxic to dogs (even small amounts).

Stevia Drops: Stevia provides various flavors including hazelnut, vanilla, English toffee, and chocolate flavors. Enjoy making a satisfying cup of sweetened coffee or other favorite drink. Some individuals think the drops are too bitter. At first, use only three drops to equal one teaspoon of sugar.

Best Types Of Butter & Oils To Use For Keto Desserts

Grass-Fed Butter: You can promote fat loss and butter is almost carb-free. The butter is a naturally occurring fatty acid that is rich in conjugated linoleic acid (CLA). It is suitable for maintaining weight loss and retaining lean muscle mass.

Ghee is also a great staple for your keto stock which is also called clarified butter.

Cashew Butter: Used in moderation, it is a healthy addition to your baking goods. The butter is usually sold in its raw form, requiring refrigeration once the package is opened. Use caution because it has 94 calories for one tbsp. as well as 8 grams of fat. Using it in moderation of no more than one or two tablespoons daily to help you feel more satisfied and fuller to help prevent you from overeating. It can provide you with potassium beta carotene, lutein, vitamin K, selenium, copper, and zinc.

Melted Coconut Oil: Coconut oil is also used as one of the best ways to improve ketone levels in people with nervous system disorders, such as those with Alzheimer's disease. The oil contains medium-chain triglycerides (MCTs) which speed up the ketosis process. Unlike many other fats, MCTs are absorbed rapidly and go directly to the liver where they are used for immediate energy – resulting in conversion to ketones.

The oil contains four types of these fats, 50% of which comes from lauric acid. Research has indicated the higher percentage may produce sustained ketosis levels because it is metabolized more gradual than other MCTs. Add coconut oil slowly to your diet because it can cause some stomach cramping or diarrhea until you adjust. Begin with one teaspoon daily, and work it up to two to three tablespoons over the span of about one week.

Avocado Oil: Avocado oil is beneficial for your blood cholesterol levels. It is high in an antioxidant (lutein) which is also a carotenoid found naturally in your eyes. You will reduce the risk of common age-related diseases while lowering the risk of cataracts.

Chapter 3: Keto Bread Recipes

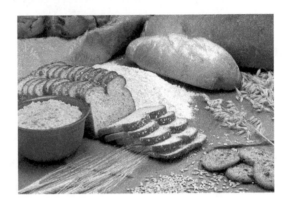

Banana Bread

Yields Provided: 16 Servings

Macro Counts For Each Serving:

- **Fat Content**: 15 g
- **Total Net Carbs**: 8 g
- **Protein**: 4 g
- **Calories**: 165

List of Ingredients:

- Bak. powder (1 tsp.)
- Xanthan gum (.5 tsp.)

- Stevia (.25 tsp.)
- Salt (.5 tsp.)
- Almond flour (.75 cup)
- Coconut flour (.33 cup)
- Vanilla extract (1 tsp.)
- Medium eggs (6)
- Erythritol (.5 cup)
- Coconut oil (3 tbsp.)
- Medium banana (1)
- Melted butter (.5 cup)

Preparation Technique:

1. Warm up the oven to reach 325° Fahrenheit.
2. Grease a loaf pan.
3. Sift or whisk the almond and coconut flour, stevia, xanthan gum, salt, erythritol, and baking powder.
4. Slice the banana, and add to a food processor with the butter, oil, eggs, and vanilla extract. Pulse for one minute and combine with the rest of the fixings. Pulse for one additional minute until well blended.
5. Empty into the pan.
6. Bake for 1 hr. 15 min. Serve when the urge strikes.

Blueberry Bread Loaf

Yields Provided: 10 Servings

Macro Counts For Each Serving:

- **Fat Content**: 17 g
- **Total Net Carbs**: 5 g
- **Protein**: 9 g
- **Calories**: 207

List of Ingredients:

- Blueberries (1 cup)
- Lemon zested (1)
- Vanilla extract (.5 tsp.)
- Lemon extract (1 tbsp.)
- Dairy-free mayonnaise (3 tbsp.)
- Medium egg whites (2)
- Whole large eggs (6)
- Salt (.25 tsp.)
- Baking soda (.5 tsp.)
- Almond flour (2 cups)
- Cream of tartar (1 tsp.)
- Coconut flour (.25 cups)
- Stevia (.75 cups)

Preparation Technique:

1. Program the oven temperature setting to reach 350° Fahrenheit.
2. Prepare the bread pan with a layer of parchment baking paper.
3. Whisk the almond flour, stevia, salt, baking soda, and coconut flour.
4. Fold in the egg whites, whole eggs, mayonnaise, lemon and vanilla extract, and lemon zest. Combine well with an electric mixer.
5. Fold in half of the berries (.5 cup) and add to the prepared pan. Bake for 20 minutes.
6. Top it off with the remainder of the berries when it is through the first baking. Continue baking for an additional 50 minutes.
7. Transfer to the counter to cool. It is best to let the bread cool for a minimum of about two hours. Serve any time.

Broccoli & Cheddar Keto Breakfast Bread

Yields Provided: 10 Servings

Macro Counts For Each Serving:

- **Fat Content**: 6 g
- **Total Net Carbs**: 1 g
- **Protein**: 6 g
- **Calories**: 90

List of Ingredients:

- Eggs (5 - beaten)
- Shredded cheddar cheese (1 cup)
- Fresh raw broccoli florets chopped (.75 cup)
- Salt (1 tsp.)
- Coconut flour (3.5 tbsp.)
- Bak. powder (2 tsp.)

Preparation Technique:

1. Heat the oven to reach 350° Fahrenheit. Spritz a loaf pan with some cooking oil spray as needed.
2. Bake for 30 to 35 minutes or until golden. Slice and serve.
3. *To Reheat The Bread*: Microwave or heat in a greased frying pan

Cauliflower Bread

Yields Provided: 10 Servings

Macro Counts For Each Serving:

- **Fat Content**: 17 g
- **Total Net Carbs**: 4 g
- **Protein**: 7 g
- **Calories**: 204

List of Ingredients:

- Riced cauliflower finely (3 cups)
- Eggs (6 large - separated)
- Olive oil (6 tbsp.)
- Super-fine almond flour (1.25 cup)
- Bak. powder (1 tbsp.)
- Salt (1 tsp.)
- _Also Needed_: 8-inch by 8-inch loaf pan

Preparation Technique:

1. Program the oven setting to 350° Fahrenheit.
2. Line the pan with parchment paper.
3. Microwave the cauliflower for 3 to 4 minutes or until tender. Let it cool, and place a small amount in a tea towel and wring dry. Repeat

with remaining cauliflower, working in small
batches.

4. Add egg whites into a bowl. Beat them until
    stiff peaks. Set aside.

5. Combine the eggs yolks, oil, baking powder,
    almond flour, and salt. Mix to form a smooth
    paste. Stir in the cauliflower until evenly
    mixed.

6. Add about ¼ of the egg whites to the paste.
    Fold in the egg whites. When the egg whites
    are completely folded in, add in another batch,
    and repeat until all of the egg whites are
    incorporated. The mixture should look pale
    and fluffy.

7. Note: Be careful not to beat the egg whites
    because that will cause them to lose the air
    whipped into them and the bread will not
    properly rise.

8. Dump the mixture into the pan. Bake for
    almost 50 minutes. Cool before slicing.

Coconut Bread

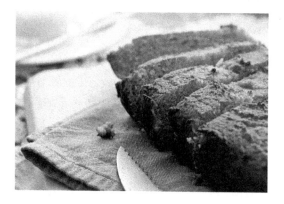

Yields Provided: 8 Servings

Macro Counts For Each Serving:

- **Fat Content:** 8.5 g
- **Total Net Carbs:** 3.8 g
- **Protein:** 9.23 g
- **Calories:** 154

List of Ingredients:

- Baking soda (.5 tsp.)
- Flaxseed meal (.5 cup)
- Baking powder (1 tsp.)
- Sifted coconut flour (1 cup)
- Salt (1 tsp.)
- Unchilled large eggs (6)
- Water (.5 cup)
- Apple cider vinegar (1 tbsp.)

Preparation Technique:

1. Warm the oven in to reach 350° Fahrenheit.
2. Lightly grease a baking pan of choice.
3. Whisk or sift the flour into a bowl and add the remainder of dry fixings. Mix well.
4. Pour in the vinegar and water to form a thick batter. Press the mixture into a prepared pan.
5. Bake until browned or for about 40 minutes.
6. Cool in the pan until slightly warm and remove. Slice and serve.

Cottage Bread

Yields Provided: 6 Servings

Macro Counts For Each Serving:

- **Fat Content**: 6.3 g
- **Total Net Carbs**: 6 g
- **Protein**: 8.4 g
- **Calories**: 109

List of Ingredients:

- Ground sesame seeds (1 tsp.)
- Ground flaxseed (1 tsp.)
- Egg (1)
- Cottage cheese (7-8 oz.)
- Turmeric powder (.125 or to taste)
- Salt (1 pinch)
- Baking powder (.5 tsp.)
- Sunflower seeds (1.5-2 oz.)
- Wheat bran (2 tbsp.)
- Oat bran (3 tbsp.)

Preparation Technique:

1. Warm up the oven to reach 425° Fahrenheit.
2. Add a sheet of parchment paper to the baking dish.

3. Combine the sesame seeds, flaxseed, egg, and cottage cheese. Shake in the salt and turmeric. Fold in the seeds, oat bran, and wheat bran.

4. Stir well and let the mixture rest for 10 minutes.

5. Shape the mixture into a ball.

6. Bake for 45 minutes in the hot oven. Remove and cool.

7. *Note:* Wet your hands with a small amount of water so the dough mixture doesn't stick to you while you prepare the bread.

Cream Cheese Bread For Rolls

Yields Provided: 6 Servings

Macro Counts For Each Serving:

- **Fat Content**: 21 g
- **Total Net Carbs**: 3 g
- **Protein**: 6 g
- **Calories**: 234

List of Ingredients:

- Baking powder (1 tsp.)
- Almond flour - blanched (1.25 cups)
- Psyllium husk powder (2-5 tbsp.)

- Celtic sea salt (1 tsp.)
- Butter (3 tbsp.)
- Boiling water (1 cup)
- Large egg (1)
- Cream cheese (4 oz.)

Preparation Technique:

1. Warm up the oven to reach 350° Fahrenheit.
2. Combine the dry components (baking powder, flour, salt, and psyllium). Set aside.
3. In another glass dish, soften the cream cheese and butter in the microwave or in a saucepan on the stove. Once it's glossy, remove from the burner/microwave and let it cool 2 minutes.
4. Add the eggs and whisk until creamy. Stir in the rest of the components to make the dough.
5. Break into small pieces and add the boiling water to firm up the dough.
6. Use a measuring cup to scoop out the dough. Place on a parchment-lined baking tin to make six rolls of bread.
7. Bake for 45 to 55 minutes and let it cool.
8. Slice the cooled bread using a serrated knife. Serve.

Dinner Rolls

Yields Provided: 6 Servings

Macro Counts For Each Serving:

- **Fat Content**: 18 g
- **Total Net Carbs**: 2.3 g
- **Protein**: 11 g
- **Calories**: 219

List of Ingredients:

- Shredded mozzarella (1 cup)
- Cream cheese (1 oz.)
- Almond flour (1 cup)
- Bak. soda (.5 tsp.)
- Ground flaxseed (.25 cup)
- Egg (1)

Preparation Technique:

1. Warm the oven to reach 400° Fahrenheit.
2. Prepare a baking pan with a sheet of parchment paper.
3. Melt the mozzarella and cream cheese together (microwave for 1 min.).
4. Stir well and add a whisked egg. Combine well.

5. In another container, whisk the baking soda, almond flour, and flaxseed. Mix in the cheese mixture to form a sticky soft-ball.

6. Dampen your hands with water and roll the dough into six balls.

7. Roll the tops in sesame seeds and move them to the baking sheet.

8. Bake (10-12 min.).

9. Cool 15 minutes and serve.

Egg Fast Cloud Bread

Yields Provided: 6 Servings

Macro Counts For Each Serving:

- **Fat Content**: 7.4 g
- **Total Net Carbs**: 0.6 g
- **Protein**: 4.2 g
- **Calories**: 85

List of Ingredients:

- Softened cream cheese (3 oz.)
- Large eggs (3)
- Salt (1 dash)
- _Optional:_ Cream of tartar preferred (1 pinch)

Preparation Technique:

1. Set the oven temperature at 300° Fahrenheit.
2. Prepare the baking pan.
3. Separate the eggs into another container.
4. Use an electric mixer to prepare the cream cheese with the salt. Add to the yolk - mixing well.
5. Whisk the cream of tartar in with the egg whites using clean mixer tongs.
6. Fold the egg yolks into the white mixture.

7. Scoop six portions onto the pan. Flatten slightly with a spatula.
8. Bake for about 24 to 30 minutes.
9. Let cool and move to the cooling rack.
10. Freeze for better results or place in a zipper-type baggie in the fridge.

Flaxseed Bread

Yields Provided: 12 Servings

Macro Counts For Each Serving:

- **Fat Content**: 7.5 g
- **Total Net Carbs**: 0.7 g
- **Protein**: 6 g
- **Calories**: 185

List of Ingredients:

- Baking powder (1 tbsp.)
- Flaxseed meal (2 cups)
- Salt (1 tsp.)
- Olive oil (.33 cup)
- Water (.5 cup)
- Whisked eggs (5)
- Maple syrup (1-2 tbsp.)
- 10 x 15-inch pan with sides

Preparation Technique:

1. Warm up the oven to 350° Fahrenheit.
2. Lightly oil a sheet of baking paper or use a mat.
3. Whisk all of the dry components. Combine with the rest of the wet components. After formed, let it rest for 2 to 3 minutes to thicken.

4. Pour into the oiled pan, pulling it away from the center for more even baking results. Stretch it into a rectangular shape, leaving about 2 inches from the end of the pan.
5. Bake until it has visible browned or 24 to 28 minutes. It is fully done when it springs back to the touch.

Delicious Buns

Garlic & Basil Buns

Yields Provided: 8 Servings

Macro Counts For Each Serving:

- **Fat Content:** 15 g
- **Total Net Carbs:** 1.4 g
- **Protein:** 9.6 g
- **Calories:** 186

List of Ingredients:

- Water (.75 cup)
- Butter (6 tbsp.)
- Salt (1 pinch)
- Chopped fresh basil (1 cup)
- Crushed garlic cloves (6)
- Eggs (4)
- Almond flour (.75 cup)
- Grated parmesan (5.5 oz)

Preparation Technique:

1. Warm up the oven to 400° Fahrenheit.
2. Cover a baking tin with a layer of parchment paper.

3. Boil the water and add the salt and butter.

4. Take the pan away from the heat and add the flour. Combine well, and break in the eggs.

5. Fold in the garlic, basil, and lastly, the parmesan.

6. Once it's creamy, add the dough on the prepared pan one spoonful at a time while shaping into buns.

7. Bake for 20 minutes and enjoy. Cool before storing.

Poppy Seed Buns

Yields Provided: 12 Servings

Macro Counts For Each Serving:

- **Fat Content**: 11.5 g
- **Total Net Carbs**: 6.2 g
- **Protein**: 10.6 g
- **Calories**: 162

List of Ingredients:

- Eggs (6 whites & 2 whole)
- Salt (.5 tsp.)
- Psyllium husk powder (.33 cup)
- Coconut flour (.5 cup)

- Almond flour (2 cups)
- Boiling water (2 cups)
- Cream of tartar (1.5 tsp.)
- Garlic powder (2 tsp.)
- Baking soda (1.3 tsp.)
- Poppy seeds (2 tbsp.)

Preparation Technique:

1. Warm up the oven to reach 350° Fahrenheit.
2. Combine all of the dry fixings.
3. In another dish, add all of the eggs and whisk. Pour in the boiling water and continue stirring.
4. Combine everything and stir until mixed well.
5. Spoon into the pan. Bake for 20 to 25 minutes.

Spring Onion Buns

Yields Provided: 6 Servings

Macro Counts For Each Serving:

- **Fat Content**: 6.7 g
- **Total Net Carbs**: 1.1 g
- **Protein**: 4.2 g
- **Calories**: 81

List of Ingredients:

- Separated eggs (3)
- Stevia (1 tsp.)
- Cream cheese (3.5 oz.)
- Baking powder (.5 tsp.)
- Salt (1 pinch)

List of Ingredients - For the Filling:

- Chopped hard-boiled egg (1)
- Diced spring onions (2 sprigs)

Preparation Technique:

1. Warm up the oven to 300° Fahrenheit.
2. Spritz the muffin cups with some oil.
3. Combine the egg yolks, stevia, cream cheese, salt, and baking powder.

4. Whisk the egg whites in another cup.

5. Combine the fixings with a spatula, and add the dough to the muffin cups.

6. Combine the filling components and add them to the cups. It is important to fill the cups only half full to allow room for the rest of the fillings.

7. Pour additional dough into the cup. Bake for 30 minutes.

8. Cool slightly and serve.

Tasty Biscuits & Focaccia

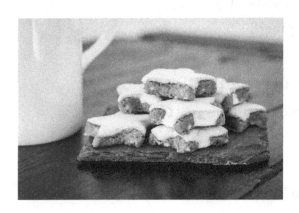

Almond Drop Biscuits With Cheese

Yields Provided: 6 Servings

Macro Counts For Each Serving:

- **Fat Content:** 13 g
- **Total Net Carbs:** 2 g
- **Protein:** 5 g
- **Calories:** 144

List of Ingredients:

- Almond flour (1.5 cups)
- Eggs (2 whole)
- Sour cream (.5 cup)
- Melted grass-fed butter (4 tbsp.)
- Shredded cheddar cheese (.5 cup)
- Swerve confectioners (1 tsp.)
- Bak. powder (1 tbsp.)
- Bak. soda (.5 tsp.)
- Salt (1 pinch)
- Cooking oil spray (as needed)

Preparation Technique:

1. Warm up the oven to reach 450° Fahrenheit.
2. Prepare a muffin pan with liners. You can also spritz the pan with a little cooking oil spray to ensure they don't stick.
3. Use a hand mixer or whisk to mix the almond flour, baking powder, salt, and baking soda.

4. Whisk eggs with the swerve, sour cream, and melted butter.
5. Combine all of the fixings.
6. Scoop the prepared batter directly into the baking pan.
7. Bake for 9 to 12 minutes.

Bacon & Cheese Drop Biscuits

Yields Provided: 10 Servings

Macro Counts For Each Serving:

- **Fat Content**: 14 g
- **Total Net Carbs**: 2 g
- **Protein**: 6 g
- **Calories**: 154

List of Ingredients:

- Almond Flour (1.5 cups)
- Onion powder (1 tsp.)
- Bak. powder (1 tbsp.)
- Bak. soda (.5 tsp.)
- Dried parsley (1 tbsp.)
- Garlic salt (1 tsp.)
- Bacon (4 slices)
- Eggs (2)
- Sour cream (.5 cup)
- Bacon grease melted (1 tbsp.)
- Shredded cheddar cheese (.33 cup)
- Shredded smoky bacon cheddar cheese (.33 cup)
- Melted grass-fed butter (3 tbsp.)

- Swerve confectioners or powdered erythritol (.5 tsp.)

Preparation Technique:

1. Set the oven temperature in advance to 425° Fahrenheit.
2. Prepare a baking pan with a layer of baking paper.
3. Cook and crumble the bacon.
4. Add the baking powder, almond flour, onion powder, garlic salt, and baking soda into a mixing container using a fork or whisk.
5. Combine the eggs, melted butter, bacon grease, bacon, parsley, sour cream.
6. Fold the cheese and combine everything.
7. Scoop the biscuit mixture onto the prepared pan.
8. Bake for 11 to 15 minutes. Serve when they are like you like them.

Biscuits & Gravy

Yields Provided: 6 Servings

Macro Counts For Each Serving:

- **Fat Content**: 60 g
- **Total Net Carbs**: 3.5 g
- **Protein**: 40 g
- **Calories**: 738

List of Ingredients - Cheddar Biscuits:

- Melted butter (.25 cup)
- Eggs (4 large)
- Coconut flour (.33 cup)
- Salt (.25 tsp.)
- Bak. powder (.25 tsp.)
- Shredded cheddar cheese (1 cup)

List of Ingredients - Gravy:

- Chicken broth (1 cup)
- Ground sausage (1 lb.)
- Heavy cream (1 cup)
- Xanthan gum (.5 tsp.)
- Black pepper & salt (as desired)

Preparation Technique:

1. Warm the oven in advance to reach 410° Fahrenheit.
2. Prepare a baking pan with a layer of parchment baking paper or spritz using a cooking oil spray.
3. Combine the biscuit fixings in a large bowl. Stir to combine.
4. Scoop 3 tbsp. worth of batter for each biscuit.
5. Arrange them two inches apart on the baking tin.
6. Bake for approximately 14 minutes. Move to the countertop.
7. Brown and crumble the sausage using the med-high heat setting until it is cooked through.
8. Pour in the chicken broth, xanthan gum, salt, pepper, and cream. Stir to combine.
9. Put it to a simmer. Continue simmering. Remove from the burner.
10. Slice the biscuits in half and spoon gravy over the biscuits.

Chapter 4: Keto Muffins

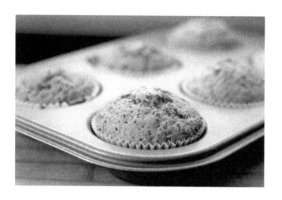

Bacon Egg Muffins

Yields Provided: 12 Servings

Macro Counts For Each Serving:

- **Fat Content:** 23.1 g
- **Total Net Carbs:** 1 g
- **Protein:** 21.5 g
- **Calories:** 300

List of Ingredients:

- Bacon (12 slices)

- Large eggs (12)
- Cheddar cheese (8 oz. grated)

Preparation Technique:

1. Heat the oven to reach 400° Fahrenheit.
2. Arrange the bacon on wire racks over a rimmed baking pan.
3. Bake for 10 to 12 minutes, removing before it's crispy.
4. Line each tin with bacon.
5. Whisk the eggs and stir in grated cheese and portion into the tin.
6. Lower the oven setting to 345° Fahrenheit. Bake for about 20 minutes until the eggs are set.
7. Transfer the muffins out of the tins and serve warm.

Banana Muffins

Yields Provided: 6 Servings

Macro Counts For Each Serving:

- **Fat Content**: 30 g
- **Total Net Carbs**: 3.5 g
- **Protein**: 8 g
- **Calories**: 332

List of Ingredients:

- Large eggs (3)
- Coconut oil (.25 cup)
- Monk fruit - 30% extract (.25 tsp.)
- Stevia powder extract (.25 tsp.)
- Coconut flour (.25 cup)
- Almond flour (.75 cup)
- Banana extract (1.75 tsp.)
- Bak. powder (1 tsp.)
- Salt (.25 tsp.)
- Cinnamon (.5 tsp.)
- Vanilla extract (1 tsp.)
- Mashed avocado (1 medium)
- Pecans (.5 cup chopped)
- *Also Needed*: 6-count muffin tin

Preparation Technique:

1. Leave the eggs out to become room temperature.
2. Warm up the oven to 350° Fahrenheit.
3. Generously grease the muffin tin.
4. Whisk the coconut oil with stevia and monk fruit.
5. Whisk in the eggs, vanilla, and banana extracts.
6. In another container, whisk or sift the coconut flour, baking powder, salt, cinnamon, and almond flour.
7. Blend into the coconut oil mixture and the mashed avocado.
8. Fold in the nuts, reserving two tablespoons to sprinkle on top.
9. Empty the batter into the molds and garnish with the nuts.
10. Bake for about 25 to 30 minutes.

Black Walnut Chocolate Chip Keto Muffins

Yields Provided: 12 Servings

Macro Counts For Each Serving:

- **Fat Content:** 26.1 g
- **Total Net Carbs:** 5.1 g
- **Protein:** 8.3 g
- **Calories:** 293

List of Ingredients:

- Almond flour (3 cups)
- Firmly packed coconut flour (4 tbsp.)
- Bak. powder (1 tbsp.)
- Salt (1 tsp.)
- Monk fruit (.75 cup)
- Bak. soda (1 tsp.)
- Melted ghee (6 tbsp.)
- Canned coconut milk - Full-fat (6 tbsp.)
- Unchilled large eggs (3)
- Vanilla extract (1 tbsp.)
- Stevia-sweetened chocolate chips (.5 cup + 1 tbsp.)
- Black walnuts (.25 cup - diced)

Preparation Technique:

1. Warm the oven to 350° Fahrenheit. Generously spritz a muffin pan with a mist of cooking oil spray.
2. Whisk or sift the almond and coconut flour, salt, baking powder, and baking soda into a mixing container.
3. Using an electric hand mixer, blend the monk fruit, coconut milk, ghee, eggs, and vanilla.
4. Stir well. Next, fold in the walnuts and chocolate chips. Let the dough rest for about five minutes so the coconut flour can begin to absorb the moisture.
5. Fill the muffin tins about two/thirds of the way to the top.
6. Bake for about 30 minutes.
7. Cool in the pan. If needed, use a butter knife around each muffin to loosen them for serving.

Blackberry-Filled Lemon Almond Flour Muffins

Yields Provided: 12 Servings

Macro Counts For Each Serving:

- **Fat Content**: 17 g
- **Total Net Carbs**: 1 g
- **Protein**: 7 g
- **Calories**: 199

List of Ingredients - The Filling:

- Granulated stevia/erythritol blend - Pyure (3 tbsp.)
- Xanthan gum (.25 tsp.)
- Water (2 tbsp.)
- Lemon juice (1 tbsp.)
- Blackberries fresh or frozen (1 cup)

List of Ingredients - The Batter:

- Super-fine almond flour (2.5 cups)
- Granulated stevia/erythritol blend (.75 cup)
- Fresh lemon zest (1 tsp.)
- Unsweetened almond milk original flavor (.25 cup)
- Butter, ghee, or coconut oil - melted (.25 cup)

- Sea salt (.5 tsp.)
- Large eggs (4)
- Grain-free baking powder (1 tsp.)
- Vanilla extract (1 tsp.)
- Lemon extract (.5 tsp.)

Preparation Technique:

1. Prepare the filling. In a 1.5 quart saucepan, whisk the granulated sweetener, and xanthan gum. Add the water, and the lemon juice one tablespoon at a time, whisking between additions.

2. Stir in the blackberries. Place the pan over the med-low heat setting. Simmer, stirring frequently. Turn the heat setting to low until the berries have broken up and a thick jammy syrup has formed (10 min.). Transfer from the heat and cool.

3. Prepare the batter. Warm the oven to 350° Fahrenheit. Prepare a muffin pan by lining with muffin papers.

4. Whisk the sea salt, almond flour, granulated sweetener, lemon zest, and baking powder.

5. Whisk the eggs, vanilla extract, almond milk, and lemon extract. Stream in butter while whisking.

6. Slowly add liquid ingredients to dry ingredients, while stirring.

7. Scoop the batter into the muffin cups. Fill about 1/3 full. Form a depression in the batter in the cups using clean fingers or a spoon.

8. Place a spoonful of the cooled blackberry jam in each depression, dividing it equally among the cups.

9. Cover the blackberry jam using the remainder of the batter until each cup is about 2/3rds full. Spread the batter to the edges of the cups to cover the jam. If cups are a little more than 2/3rds full after all of the batters are used up, that's okay.

10. Bake for 30 minutes. Refrigerate any extras in an airtight container. They may also be frozen if desired.

Blueberry Cream Cheese Muffins

Yields Provided: 12 Servings

Macro Counts For Each Serving:

- **Fat Content**: 14 g
- **Total Net Carbs**: 2 g
- **Protein**: 3 g
- **Calories**: 154

List of Ingredients:

- Softened unchilled cream cheese (16 oz.)
- Low-carb sweetener (.5 cup)
- Eggs (2)
- Xanthan gum optional (.25 tsp.)
- Sugar-free vanilla extract (.5 tsp.)
- Blueberries (.25 cup)
- Sliced almonds (.25 cup)
- _Also Needed_: 12-count muffin molds with paper liners

Preparation Technique:

1. Set the oven temperature to 345° Fahrenheit.
2. Blend the cheese until it's smooth.
3. Stir in the eggs, vanilla, sweetener, and xanthan gum.

71

4. Mix well. Stir in the blueberries and almonds.

5. Scoop into the molds and bake for about 20 minutes.

6. Chill and serve.

Brownie Pumpkin Muffins

Yields Provided: 6 Servings

Macro Counts For Each Serving:

- **Fat Content:** 13 g
- **Total Net Carbs:** 4.4 g
- **Protein:** 7 g
- **Calories:** 183

List of Ingredients:

- Salt (.5 tsp.)
- Flaxseed meal (1 cup)
- Cocoa powder (.25 cup)
- Cinnamon (1 tbsp.)
- Baking powder (.5 tbsp.)
- Coconut oil (2 tbsp.)
- Large egg (1)
- Sugar-free caramel syrup (.25 cup)
- Vanilla extract (1 tsp.)
- Pumpkin puree (.5 cup)
- Slivered almonds (.5 cup)
- Apple cider vinegar (1 tsp.)

Preparation Technique:

1. Set the oven temperature at 350° Fahrenheit.

2. Combine each of the fixings and stir well.

3. Use six paper liners in the muffin tin, and add .25 cup of batter into each one. Sprinkle several almonds on the tops, pressing gently.

4. Bake approximately 15 minutes or when the top is set.

Chocolate Chip & Peanut Butter Mini Muffins

Yields Provided: 24 Servings

Macro Counts For Each Serving:

- **Fat Content**: 9.8 g
- **Total Net Carbs**: 4.3 g
- **Protein**: 8.1 g
- **Calories**: 130

List of Ingredients:

- Peanut flour (1 cup)
- Salt (.25 tsp.)
- Bak. powder (1.5 tsp.)
- Peanut butter (.33 cup)
- Golden low carb sweetener or other brown sugar replacement (.33 cup)
- Butter/coconut oil (2 tbsp.)
- Large egg (1)
- Almond milk or coconut milk (.33 cup)
- Sugar-free chocolate chips (.25 cup)

Preparation Technique:

1. In advance, set the oven temperature to reach 350° Fahrenheit.

2. Prepare the (24- count) mini muffin pan with baking cups.

3. Sift the salt with the peanut flour and baking powder.

4. In another container; mix the peanut butter, butter, and sweetener until creamy.

5. Fold in the whisked egg and milk until smooth.

6. Combine everything until blended.

7. Lastly, add in the chocolate chips.

8. Scoop the batter into the cups using a cookie scoop for convenience.

9. Bake for 10-12 minutes.

10. Set to the side and cool for about five minutes

Chocolate Zucchini Muffins - Sugar-Free

Yields Provided: 12 Servings

Macro Counts For Each Serving:

- **Fat Content:** 15.9 g
- **Total Net Carbs:** 2.4 g
- **Protein:** 3.8 g
- **Calories:** 179

List of Ingredients:

- Eggs (5)
- Erythritol (.75 cup)
- Salt (.5 tsp.)
- Cocoa powder - unsweetened (3 tbsp.)
- Vanilla extract (.75 cup)
- Almond flour (1 cup)
- Baking soda (.5 tsp.)
- Shredded zucchini (1 cup)
- Coconut oil or Melted butter (.5 cup)
- Coconut flour (.5 cup)
- Baking powder (.5 tsp.)
- Cinnamon (.5 tsp.)
- *Also Needed:* Cooking oil spray & 12-count muffin baking mold

Preparation Technique:

1. Set the oven temperature at 330° Fahrenheit.
2. Lightly spritz the muffin molds with some cooking oil spray.
3. Mix the sweetener and butter or oil.
4. Whisk and add in the eggs; adding the vanilla, zucchini, and cocoa.
5. In another container, combine all of the fixings and add the batter to the molds.
6. Bake around 30 min.
7. *Note*: Omit the salt if using salted butter.
8. Transfer the muffins from the molds to cool on a wire rack.
9. When cooled, place in a covered container in the fridge until needed.

Cinnamon Applesauce Muffins

Yields Provided: 12 Servings

Macro Counts For Each Serving:

- **Fat Content:** 22 g
- **Total Net Carbs:** 3 g
- **Protein:** 7 g
- **Calories:** 240

List of Ingredients:

- Melted ghee (.5 cup)
- Large whisked eggs (3)
- Nutmeg (1 tsp.)
- Cinnamon (3 tbsp.)
- Cloves (.25 tsp.)
- Applesauce (4 tbsp.)
- Bak. powder (1 tsp.)
- Stevia (to your liking)
- Almond flour (3 cups)
- Lemon juice (1 tsp.)

Preparation Technique:

1. Program the oven temperature setting to 350° Fahrenheit.
2. Combine the fixings in a mixing container.
3. Move the batter into pan.
4. Bake for 20 min.
5. Cool.

Cinnamon Roll Muffins

Yields Provided: 20 Servings

Macro Counts For Each Serving:

- **Fat Content**: 9 g
- **Total Net Carbs**: 3 g
- **Protein**: 5 g
- **Calories**: 112

List of Ingredients:

- Almond flour (.5 cup)
- Vanilla protein powder (2 scoops)
- Cinnamon (1 tbsp.)
- Bak. powder (1 tsp.)
- Nut or seed butter of choice (.5 cup)
- Pumpkin puree or unsweetened applesauce, mashed cooked sweet potato, or mashed banana (.5 cup)
- Coconut oil (.5 cup)
- Also Needed: 12-count muffin tin

List of Ingredients - For the Glaze:

- Coconut butter (.25 cup)
- Granulated sweetener of choice (1 tbsp.)
- Milk -your favorite (.25 cup)
- Lemon juice (2 tsp.)

Preparation Technique:

1. Warm the oven to 345° Fahrenheit and prepare the tin with muffin liners.
2. Combine the dry fixings and mix well. Mix in the wet ones until fully incorporated.
3. Empty the batter into the cups.
4. Bake for 12 to 15 minutes, checking around the 10-minute mark by inserting a skewer in the center and seeing if it comes out clean. Cool.
5. Once cooled, prepare your cinnamon roll glaze by combining all of the ingredients and mixing until combined. Drizzle over the muffin tops and cool to firm up.

Chapter 5: Keto Cookies

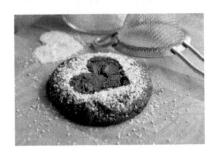

Butter Cookies

Yields Provided: 10 Servings

Macro Counts For Each Serving:

- **Fat Content**: 9 g
- **Total Net Carbs**: 1 g
- **Protein**: 2 g
- **Calories**: 100

List of Ingredients:

- Blanched almond flour (1 cup)
- Powdered erythritol (.25 cup) or Confectioners swerve (3 tbsp.)
- Unchilled salted butter (3 tbsp.)
- Vanilla extract (.5 tsp.)

Preparation Technique:

1. Warm to 345°.
2. Prepare a sheet lined with a layer of baking paper.
3. Combine all of the fixings, stirring to form a dough.
4. Work the dough to form ten 1-inch balls, placing them on the baking sheet about 2 inches apart.
5. Flatten each dough ball, form a crisscross pattern using a fork. Note that these cookies will maintain their shape during baking and won't spread.
6. Bake about 12 minutes depending on the thickness of the cookies.
7. Cool completely before removing from the baking sheet.

Butter Pecan Cookies

Yields Provided: 20 Servings

Macro Counts For Each Serving:

- **Fat Content**: 22.3 g
- **Total Net Carbs**: 2.2 g
- **Protein**: 5 g
- **Calories**: 240

List of Ingredients:

- Unsalted butter softened (.5 cup)
- Swerve Sweetener (.5 cup)
- Almond flour (1.75 cups)
- Salt (.5 tsp.)
- Coconut flour (2 tbsp.)
- Vanilla extract (.5 tsp.)
- Chopped toasted pecans (.5 cup)

Preparation Technique:

1. Set the oven at 325° Fahrenheit. Prepare two rimmed baking tins with a layer of parchment baking paper.
2. Beat the butter and sweetener together until fluffy (2 min.).
3. Mix in coconut flour, almond flour, salt, vanilla extract, and chopped pecans.

4. Roll the dough into one-inch balls. Arrange a few inches apart in the cookie sheets. Flatten slightly.
5. Bake for 5 minutes. Remove from the oven and flatten again to about ¼-inch thickness. Bake another 10 to 12 minutes.
6. Remove and cool.

Chocolate Fudge Keto Cookies

Yields Provided: 10 Servings

Macro Counts For Each Serving:

- **Fat Content:** 11.6 g
- **Total Net Carbs:** 2 g
- **Protein:** 4.4 g
- **Calories:** 132

List of Ingredients:

- Swerve confectioner (.5 cup)
- Unsweetened cocoa powder (.5 cup)
- Butter (.25 cup)
- Eggs (2 large)
- Bak. powder (1 tsp.)
- Almond flour (1 cup)
- Pink Himalayan Salt (1 pinch)
- Vanilla extract (1 tsp.)
- Optional: Erythritol as desired

Preparation Technique:

1. Whisk the cocoa powder and swerve confectioners' sugar in a mixing bowl. Melt and add the butter, mixing with a hand mixer.

2. Once combined, add eggs, vanilla, and baking powder. Mix again.

3. Add the almond flour and mix one last time.

4. Form into cookies and place on a greased cookie sheet. The cookies will remain the shape you form them to after cooking.

5. Dust the tops of cookies with erythritol.

6. Bake at 355° Fahrenheit for 13-15 minutes. Cool and serve.

Chocolate Sea Salt Cookies

Yields Provided: 15 Servings

Macro Counts For Each Serving:

- **Fat Content:** 18.2 g
- **Total Net Carbs:** 1.6 g
- **Protein:** 3.4g
- **Calories:** 188

List of Ingredients:

- Unchilled coconut oil (.75 cup)
- Eggs (2)
- Vanilla extract (1 tsp.)
- Golden monk fruit sweetener (.75 cup)
- Unsweetened cocoa powder (2 tbsp.)
- Salt (.5 tsp.)
- Cream of tartar (.25 tsp.)
- Bak. soda (.5 tsp.)
- Almond flour (2 cups)
- Flaky sea salt (as desired)

Preparation Technique:

1. Warm the oven in advance to baking to reach 355° Fahrenheit.

2. Set up two baking sheets with a layer of parchment baking paper.
3. Prepare using a hand mixer. Combine the eggs, coconut oil, and vanilla extract.
4. Toss in the baking soda, cocoa powder, salt, sweetener, and cream of tartar. Mix thoroughly.
5. Gradually fold in the almond flour.
6. Form the dough into balls. Place the dough onto the baking sheet. Arrange the balls about two to three inches apart.
7. Garnish using sea salt a top of each cookie.
8. Bake the cookies for about 16 to 20 minutes; baking one tray at a time.
9. Remove and cool completely.
10. Gently pull the paper away from each of the cookies. Serve.

Cinnamon Walnut Cookies

Yields Provided: 16 Servings

Macro Counts For Each Serving:

- **Fat Content:** 7 g
- **Total Net Carbs:** 1 g
- **Protein:** 3 g
- **Calories:** 72

List of Ingredients:

- Ground walnuts (1.5 cups)
- Ground cinnamon (1 tsp.)
- Erythritol (2 tbsp.)
- Egg (1)

Preparation Technique:

1. Set the oven temperature to reach 350° Fahrenheit. Cover a cookie tray with parchment paper.
2. Finely grind the nuts, leaving medium-sized pieces to your liking.
3. Combine the cinnamon and erythritol with the egg. Fold in the walnuts.
4. Shape into balls and arrange onto the cookie tin.
5. Bake for 10 to 13 minutes.

Easy Sugar Cookies

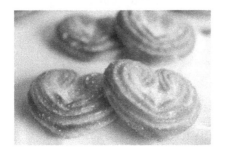

Yields Provided: 24 Servings

Macro Counts For Each Serving:

- **Total Net Carbs**: 0.8 g
- **Fat Content**: 5.4 g
- **Protein**: 1.6 g
- **Calories**: 59.2

List of Ingredients:

- Unchilled butter (5 tbsp.)
- Monkfruit Sweetener (.5 cup)
- Unchilled egg (1 large)
- Pure almond extract (.5 tsp.)
- Pure vanilla extract (1 tsp.)
- Almond flour (1.25 cups)
- Packed coconut flour (4 tbsp.)
- Baking Powder (.5 tsp.)
- Salt (.25 tsp.)

Preparation Technique:

1. Use an electric hand mixer and cream the butter and monk fruit until well combined. Mix in the egg and extracts. Beat on high speed until fluffy.
2. Add all the remaining fixings into the bowl and stir until well mixed.
3. Form the cookie dough into a disc, wrapping tightly using plastic cling wrap. Pop in the fridge for at least six hours, but it's best overnight.
4. Once chilled, warm the oven to 380° Fahrenheit. Cover a cookie sheet with a layer of parchment baking paper.
5. Roll the cookie dough between 2 large pieces of parchment ** (one piece under the cookie dough and one on top of it, under the rolling pin) to reach .25-inch thickness. Cut into shaped cookies and arrange them on the prepared pan.
6. Bake until the edges are lightly golden brown (10-11 min.). They firm up a lot once cool.
7. Let cool completely.

Chapter 6: Keto Bagels

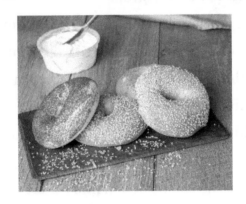

Almond Fathead Bagels

Yields Provided: 6 Servings

Macro Counts For Each Serving:

- **Fat Content**: 31 g
- **Total Net Carbs**: 5 g
- **Protein**: 20 g
- **Calories**: 377

List of Ingredients:

- Almond flour (1.5 cups)
- Mozzarella cheese (2.5 cups)
- Cream cheese (3 oz.)
- Eggs (2)
- Egg white - beaten with a little water (1)

- Baking powder (1 tbsp.)
- Salt (.25 tsp.)
- Flavorless oil (1 tsp.)
- *Optional:* Everything Bagel Seasoning
- *Optional:* Sesame seeds

Preparation Technique:

1. Set the oven temperature to 400° Fahrenheit.
2. Prepare a baking sheet using a sheet of baking paper.
3. Toss the mozzarella and cream cheese in the microwave-safe container.
4. Set the timer for one minute and set aside for now.
5. Sift the almond flour, salt, and baking powder in a mixing dish. Whisk and add in one of the eggs.
6. Shred the mozzarella and fold in with the cream cheese.
7. Portion the dough into six balls. Poke your finger in the middle and work it to form the shape.
8. Arrange the bagels on a baking sheet.
9. Whisk an egg and gently brush the tops. Leave plain or add your favorite toppings.

10. Bake for approximately 13 to 15 minutes. The tops will have browned to your liking.
11. Serve with a portion of butter or cream cheese.
12. Note: As the cheese cools, it may become more difficult to mix. You can microwave the dough for 10 seconds to make it more pliable.

Asiago Bagels

Yields Provided: 8 Servings

Macro Counts For Each Serving:
- **Fat Content**: 21 g
- **Total Net Carbs**: 6 g
- **Protein**: 20 g
- **Calories**: 293

List of Ingredients:
- Shredded mozzarella (2 cups)
- Shredded asiago (1 cup)
- Cream cheese (.25 cup)
- Free-range eggs (2)
- Organic almond flour (1.5 cups)
- Gluten-free baking powder (1 tbsp.)
- Sea salt (.5 tsp.)

Preparation Technique:

1. Heat the oven to reach 400° Fahrenheit. Mix the almond flour, eggs, baking powder, and salt.

2. Melt the mozzarella and cheese in Microwave. Combine the melted cheese mixture, almond flour, and 3/4 cup shredded asiago. It will be very thick and dough-like.

3. Working with your hands, shape into a ball and knead until each of the fixings is thoroughly combined.

4. Break the dough into eight pieces and shape each into a ball. Poke holes in the middle to make bagel shapes.

5. Sprinkle the 1/4 cup of asiago cheese on the bagels. Arrange on a sheet pan and bake for 20 min.

6. Add your favorite bagel toppings.

Bacon Breakfast Bagels

Yields Provided: 3 Servings

Macro Counts For Each Serving:

- **Fat Content**: 50.29 g
- **Total Net Carbs**: 5.76 g
- **Protein**: 30.13 g
- **Calories**: 605.7

List of Ingredients - The Bagels:

- Almond flour (.75 cup)
- Xanthan gum (1 tsp.)
- Grated mozzarella (1.5 cups)
- Cream cheese (2 tbsp.)
- Large egg (1)

List of Ingredients - The Fillings:

- Cream cheese (2 tbsp.)
- Arugula leaves (1 cup)
- Pesto (2 tbsp.)
- Grilled sliced bacon (6)
-

List of Ingredients - The Toppings:

- Melted butter (1 tbsp.)
- Sesame seeds (to your liking)

Preparation Technique:

1. Set the temperature in the oven to 380° Fahrenheit.
2. Mix the xanthan gum, almond flour, and egg until well mixed. Set aside.
3. Melt the cream cheese and mozzarella and mix it into the almond flour mix. Knead well.
4. Split the dough into three segments and roll into round logs. Place in a donut pan or a baking tin.
5. Brush melted butter over the tops of the bagels. Sprinkle with the desired toppings such as seeds, garlic or onion powder for a savory flavor.
6. Bake for 18-20 minutes. Then cool.
7. Slice and place back in the oven until slightly golden and toasty. Spread with cream cheese, pesto, and a few arugula leaves. Garnish with crispy bacon.

Cauliflower Everything Bagel

Yields Provided: 4 Servings (2 pieces)

Macro Counts For Each Serving:

- **Fat Content:** 11 g
- **Total Net Carbs:** 6 g
- **Protein:** 11 g
- **Calories:** 185

List of Ingredients:

- Cauliflower florets (about 1.5 lb./6 cups)
- Shredded sharp cheddar cheese (1 cup)
- Large egg (1)
- Everything Bagel Seasoning (2.5 tsp.)

Preparation Technique:

1. Set the oven temperature at 425° Fahrenheit. Cover a baking tin using a layer of parchment baking paper.
2. Toss the cauliflower into a food processor to finely chop and dump into a microwave-safe bowl. Microwave for 3 min.
3. Remove the moisture from the cauliflower. Mix in the egg and cheddar cheese.

4. Divide into eight portions on the baking sheet. Make a hole in the center to form the bagels. Sprinkle with seasoning.
5. Bake for at least 22 minutes.
6. Prepare in advance if desired.

Cheesy Keto Bagels

Yields Provided: 6 Servings

Macro Counts For Each Serving:

- **Fat Content**: 27.9 g
- **Total Net Carbs**: 5.9 g
- **Protein**: 22.8 g
- **Calories**: 356

List of Ingredients:

- Almond flour (1.5 cups)
- Coconut flour (3 tbsp.)
- Cream of tartar (2 tsp.)
- Bak. soda (1 tsp.)
- Shredded mozzarella (2.5 cups)
- Cream cheese (2 oz.)
- Large eggs (3)
- Sesame seeds (2 tsp.)

Preparation Technique:

1. Warm up the oven to reach 400°.
2. Prepare a layer of paper
3. Sift the coconut flour, almond flour, cream of tartar, and baking soda.

4. Add the shredded mozzarella and cream cheese into a safe dish, and microwave for 90 seconds. Remove the dish and stir.
5. Return to microwave and cook for one more minute until they're completely combined.
6. Whisk two eggs and add to the dry fixings.
7. Add melted cheese mixture into the bowl of flour and eggs. Knead the dough until all ingredients are incorporated. Divide the dough into six portions.
8. Gently roll each of the portions into a log shape attach the two ends to make the log into the bagel circle. Arrange the dough on the paper-lined baking sheet.
9. Whisk the remaining egg and gently brush the egg wash over the tops. Sprinkle the sesame seeds on top.
10. Bake the bagels until golden brown (15 min.).
11. Move the pan of bagels from the oven. Be sure to cool for at least 15 minutes for the best results.
12. Once they are cool, just store in a closed container.

Cinnamon Sugar Bagels

Yields Provided: 6 Servings

Macro Counts For Each Serving:

- **Fat Content:** 19.9 g
- **Total Net Carbs:** 5.6 g
- **Protein:** 25.4g
- **Calories:** 317

List of Ingredients:

- Almond flour (1.75 cups)
- Cream of tartar (2 tsp.)
- Coconut flour (.25 cup)
- Baking soda (1 tsp.)
- Golden monk fruit sweetener - divided (3 tbsp.)
- Cinnamon - divided (1 tbsp.)
- Shredded mozzarella (2.5 cups)
- Cream cheese (2 oz.)
- Large eggs (3)

Preparation Technique:

1. Program the oven temperature setting to reach 400° Fahrenheit.

2. Prepare a baking sheet using a layer of parchment baking paper.

3. Whisk one tablespoon of the monk fruit sweetener, coconut flour, baking soda, almond flour, cream of tartar, and one teaspoon of cinnamon.

4. Add the mozzarella and cream cheese into a microwave-safe bowl. Cook for 90 seconds. Remove the dish carefully and stir the fixings.

5. Return to cook for another minute. Stir well to combine.

6. In another container, whisk two eggs, and add to the large container of flour. Pour the cheese mixture in with the eggs and flour. Knead the dough and divide into 6 portions, connecting the two ends to create the bagels. Place onto the sheet.

7. In another container, whisk the last egg. Using a pastry brush, cover each of the bagels. Mix the cinnamon and remainder of the sweetener to sprinkle over the tops.

8. Bake for 13 to 14 minutes.

9. When ready, cool for a minimum of 15/20 minutes.

Coconut Fathead Butter Bagels

Yields Provided: 2 Servings

Macro Counts For Each Serving:

- **Fat Content**: 16 g
- **Total Net Carbs**: 4 g
- **Protein**: 14 g
- **Calories**: 234

List of Ingredients:

- Coconut flour (.5 cup)
- Aluminum-free baking powder (2 tbsp.)
- Cream cheese (2 oz.)
- Shredded mozzarella cheese (2.5 cups)
- Melted butter (2 tbsp.)

Preparation Technique:

1. Program the oven temperature setting to 410° Fahrenheit.
2. Prepare a baking pan with a layer of baking paper.
3. Whisk or sift the coconut flour and baking powder into a mixing container.

4. Melt the mozzarella and cheese for 1 minute using high power in the microwave. Stir and cook for another minute.
5. Mix in the beaten eggs, butter, and coconut flour mixture to form the dough.
6. Divide the dough into six segments. Roll and form the bagel.
7. Place the bagels on the baking tin. Bake until lightly browned (approx. 12 to 16 min.). Serve.

Coconut Flour Garlic Bagels

Yields Provided: 6 Servings

Macro Counts For Each Serving:

- **Fat Content**: 16 g
- **Total Net Carbs**: 3 g
- **Protein**: 8 g
- **Calories**: 191

List of Ingredients:

- Melted butter (.33 cup)
- Sifted coconut flour (.5 cup)
- Bak. powder (.5 tsp.)
- Guar gum or xanthan gum - optional (2 tsp.)
- Eggs (6)
- Salt (.5 tsp.)
- Garlic powder (1.5 tsp.)
- Also Needed: Donut pan

Preparation Technique:

1. Set the oven at 400° Fahrenheit.
2. Lightly grease the pan.
3. Blend together eggs, butter, salt, and garlic powder.

4. Combine coconut flour with baking powder and guar or xanthan gum.
5. Whisk the coconut flour mixture into the batter until there are no lumps.
6. Scoop into the pan. Bake for 15 minutes.
7. Cool on a rack for 10-15 minutes.
8. Transfer the bagels from the pan to cool or serve.
9. Store in the fridge.

Chapter 7: Keto Pizza

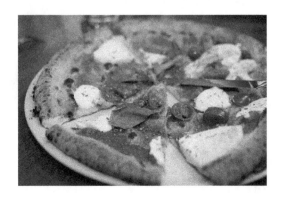

Almond Flour Pizza Crust & Topping

Yields Provided: 4 Servings - 2 Slices each

Macro Counts For Each Serving:

- **Fat Content**: 37 g
- **Total Net Carbs**: 8 g
- **Protein**: 24 g
- **Calories**: 466

List of Ingredients:

- Kosher salt(1 tsp.)
- Blanched almond flour (2 cups)
- Bak. soda (1 tsp.)
- Garlic powder (1 tsp.)
- Large egg (1)

List of Ingredients – The Topping:

- Rao's pizza sauce or keto-friendly option (.5 cup)
- Shredded part-skim mozzarella cheese (6 oz. or 1.5 cups)

Preparation Technique:

1. Set the oven ahead of time to reach 400° Fahrenheit. Prepare a sheet with a layer of baking paper.
2. Whisk the kosher salt, baking soda, almond flour, and garlic powder.
3. Whisk the egg and mix it into the flour mixture. Knead with the dry fixings to prepare into a smooth dough.
4. Transfer the dough into the prepared baking pan. Roll into a large (¼-inch-thick circle) 10-inch diameter with a rolling pin.
5. Bake for 7-8 minutes. Remove the crust from the oven and increase the temperature to broil. Set a rack six inches below flame.
6. Top the crust with the pizza sauce, mozzarella, and other toppings of choice. If needed, you can cover the edges of the crust with strips of foil to prevent them from scorching.

7. Broil the pizza briefly (2-3 min.). Cool and wait for five minutes before serving.

Breakfast Keto Pizza

Yields Provided: 2 Servings

Macro Counts For Each Serving:

- **Fat Content**: 31 g
- **Total Net Carbs**: 8.8 g
- **Protein**: 22 g
- **Calories**: 454

List of Ingredients:

- Grated cauliflower (2 cups)
- Coconut flour (2 tbsp.)
- Salt (.5 tsp.)
- Eggs (4)
- Psyllium husk powder (1 tbsp.)
- _Toppings_: Smoked salmon, avocado, herbs, spinach, olive oil, etc.

Preparation Technique:

1. Warm the oven to 350° Fahrenheit. Cover a pizza tray with parchment baking paper.
2. Add all of the fixings except toppings. Mix until combined. Set aside for about five minutes to thicken.

3. Carefully pour the breakfast pizza base onto the pan. Use your hands to mold it into a round, even pizza crust.

4. Bake or until golden brown and fully cooked (15 min.).

5. Remove from the oven and top breakfast pizza with your chosen toppings. Serve warm.

Breakfast Pizza Waffles

Yields Provided: 2 Servings

Macro Counts For Each Serving:

- **Fat Content**: 48 g
- **Total Net Carbs**: 7.6 g
- **Protein**: 30.7g
- **Calories**: 604

List of Ingredients:

- Large eggs (4)
- Italian seasoning (1 tsp.)
- Psyllium husk powder (1 tbsp.)
- Almond flour (3 tbsp.)
- Baking powder (1 tsp.)
- Salt and pepper (as desired)
- Bacon grease (1 tbsp.)
- Tomato sauce (.5 cup)
- Cheddar cheese (3 oz.)
- Grated parmesan cheese (4 tbsp.)
- _Optional_: Pepperoni (14 slices)

Preparation Technique:

1. Prepare using an immersion blender to mix all of the fixings until it thickens (omit the tomato sauce and cheese).

2. Heat the waffle iron. Prepare the batter in two batches.

3. Add the tomato sauce (.25 cup each) and cheese (1.5 oz. each) onto each waffle.

4. Broil for three to five minutes in the oven. Add pepperoni as desired but add the carbs.

Cauliflower Pizza Crust

Yields Provided: 8 Servings

Macro Counts For Each Serving:

- **Fat Content**: 6 g
- **Total Net Carbs**: 3 g
- **Protein**: 10 g
- **Calories**: 106

List of Ingredients:

- Large egg (1)
- Cauliflower florets (1.5 cups)
- Grated parmesan cheese (1.5 cups)

List Of Optional Ingredients:

- Italian seasoning (.5 tbsp.)
- Garlic powder (.5 tsp.)

Preparation Technique:

1. Set the oven temperature at 400° Fahrenheit.
2. Prepare a pizza pan or stone and line it with a sheet of parchment paper.
3. Pulse the florets in a food processor to make riced cauliflower. On the stovetop, sauté the florets for about 10 minutes until softened.

4. Whisk the egg and blend in with the cheese and seasonings (if using).
5. Pour the rice into the mixture. Mix well and press with a spatula. (It is much easier to prepare two small pizzas.)
6. Spread the dough into the pan until about .25-inch thick. Bake until browned and firm (20 min.).
7. Let the crust cool a minimum of 5 to 10 minutes at room temperature. Add toppings. Put it back to the oven and let the cheese melt.

Chewy Low-Carb Pizza Crust

Yields Provided: 6 Servings

Macro Counts For Each Serving:

- **Fat Content:** 20 g
- **Total Net Carbs:** 2 g
- **Protein:** 18 g
- **Calories:** 268

List of Ingredients:

- Shredded mozzarella cheese (1.5 cups)
- Pinch of salt (1 pinch)
- Garlic powder (.5 tsp.)
- Grated parmesan cheese (2 tbsp.)
- Hemp seeds (.75 cup)
- Baking powder (.5 tsp.)
- Eggs (3)

Preparation Technique:

1. Set the oven to 350° Fahrenheit.
2. Add a layer of parchment baking paper onto a baking sheet.
3. Combine all of the fixings, stirring well.
4. Let sit for about 5 minutes.

5. Using a 1/4 cup measure, make six mounds of cheese mixture on the baking sheet. Pat down to about .25-inch thickness.

6. Bake for 20 minutes. Cool before removing from pans.

Chicken Crust Pizza

Yields Provided: 8 Servings

Macro Counts For Each Serving:

- **Fat Content**: 13 g
- **Total Net Carbs**: 0.8 g
- **Protein**: 14 g
- **Calories**: 172

List of Ingredients:

- Chicken thighs (1 lb.)
- Shredded mozzarella - whole milk (1 cup)
- Large egg (1)
- Dried oregano (1 tsp.)
- Black pepper and salt (.25 tsp. each)
- Butter (2 tbsp.)
- Celery (1 stalk)
- Sour cream (1 tbsp.)
- Franks Red Hot Original (3 tbsp.)
- Blue cheese crumbles (1 oz.)
- Green onion (1 stalk)

Preparation Technique:

1. Set the oven temperature to 400° Fahrenheit. Cut and place a sheet of parchment paper onto a pizza pan and set aside.
2. Remove all of the bones and skin from the chicken. Grind using the blade attachment on a food processor into a large mixing container. Finely dice the celery.
3. Whisk and add the egg, salt, and .5 cup of shredded mozzarella to the mixing container.
4. Mix the crust until all of the shredded cheese is enclosed in the dough.
5. Spread the chicken out until it's .25-inch thick in the pizza pan. Bake until the crust is starting to brown on top (25 min.).
6. Meanwhile, add and melt the butter in a skillet and sauté the celery until it wilts.
7. Blend in 2 tbsp. of hot sauce and sour cream.
8. Remove the crust and add the sauce layered with the celery, rest of the mozzarella, and crumbles of blue cheese.
9. Bake until the cheese is melted (10 min.). Switch to broil for the last few minutes.
10. Drizzle hot sauce and garnish with green onion slices before serving.

Crunchy Cheese Pizza

Yields Provided: 4 Servings (2 slices each)

Macro Counts For Each Serving:

- **Fat Content:** 23 g
- **Total Net Carbs:** 1 g
- **Protein:** 19 g
- **Calories:** 298

List of Ingredients:

- Pepperoni (2 oz.)
- Mushrooms (3)
- Oregano (2 pinch - dried)
- Keto-friendly marinara sauce (2 tbsp.)
- Shredded cheddar cheese (.5 cup)
- Mozzarella cheese (2 cups)
- Also Needed: High-heat non-stick skillet

Preparation Technique:

1. Thinly slice the pepperoni and mushrooms and toss onto a lined cookie sheet. Broil/grill for 3 to 5 minutes.
2. Place the pan using the high-heat temperature setting. Spread the mozzarella cheese evenly over the pan, then sprinkle over the cheddar.

Work the cheese in off the edges of the pan. Sprinkle over the oregano.

3. Spread the marinara sauce around the melting cheese, try not to work it down into the cheese rather over it.

4. Add the pepperoni and mushrooms.

5. When the base is golden brown, crispy and begins to lift as one piece, your pizza is ready.

6. Carefully slide the pizza off onto a chopping board or cutting surface and cut into 8 equal pieces.

7. Serve.

Fathead Pizza Crust

Yields Provided: 8 Servings

Macro Counts For Each Serving:

- **Fat Content:** 8 g
- **Total Net Carbs:** 2 g
- **Protein:** 7 g
- **Calories:** 117

List of Ingredients:

- Shredded mozzarella cheese (1.5 cups
- Cubed cream cheese (2 tbsp.)
- Large eggs (2 beaten)
- Coconut flour (.33 cup)

Preparation Technique:

1. Warm the oven to reach 425° Fahrenheit).
2. Prepare a pizza pan with a sheet of parchment baking paper.
3. Toss the shredded mozzarella and cubed cream cheese into a large mixing container. Microwave for 90 seconds, stirring halfway through. Stir again.
4. Stir in the whisked eggs and coconut flour. Knead with your hands to form the dough.

5. Spread the dough onto the lined baking pan to ¼-inch or ⅓-inch thickness, using your hands or a rolling pin over a piece of parchment. Poke air holes throughout the crust to prevent bubbling.
6. Bake for 6 minutes.

Chapter 8: Sweets & Snacks

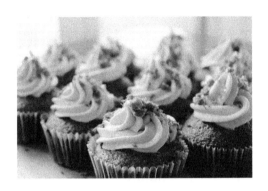

Baked Apples

Yields Provided: 4 Servings

Macro Counts For Each Serving:

- **Fat Content**: 33 g
- **Total Net Carbs**: 7 g
- **Protein**: 4 g
- **Calories**: 345

List of Ingredients:

- Unchilled butter (2 oz.)
- Walnuts/Pecans (1 oz.)

- Coconut flour (4 tbsp.)
- Ground cinnamon (.5 tsp.)
- Vanilla extract (.25 tsp.)
- Sour/tart apple (1)

For Serving:
- Heavy whipping cream (.75 cup)
- Vanilla extract (.5 tsp.)

Preparation Technique:

1. Warm the oven to reach 350° Fahrenheit. Lightly spritz a baking dish.
2. Mix the softened butter, cinnamon, coconut flour, chopped nuts, and vanilla into a crumbly dough.
3. Cut both ends off of the apple and slice into four pieces; leaving the peel and seeds are okay. Arrange the slices in the baking dish and sprinkle the dough crumbs.
4. Bake for 15 minutes.
5. Pour the heavy whipping cream and vanilla into a mixing container. Whisk briskly until soft peaks are created.
6. Slightly cool the apples and enjoy with a portion of the whipped cream.

Baked Brie With Almonds

Yields Provided: 8 Servings

Macro Counts For Each Serving:

- **Fat Content**: 25 g
- **Total Net Carbs**: 4 g
- **Protein**: 17 g
- **Calories**: 323

List of Ingredients:

- Cream cheese (2 oz.)
- Cubed or shredded mozzarella (8 oz.)
- Egg (1)
- Bak. powder (1 tsp.)
- Almond flour (.33 cup)
- Coconut flour (.33 cup)
- Ground golden flax (.33 cup)

List of Ingredients - The Assembly:

- Round brie (8 oz.) **
- Sugar-free cranberry sauce (.25 cup)
- Sliced almonds (.25 cup)
- Truvia or sweetener of your choice (1 tbsp.)

Preparation Technique:

1. Set the oven temperature at 400° Fahrenheit.

2. Toss the cheese into a microwave-safe bowl to melt for one minute. Stir. Microwave another 30 seconds and add the rest of the dough into a food processor. Mix using the dough blade.

3. Arrange the dough on a layer of parchment baking paper (a little wider than the brie). Put the cranberry sauce in the middle of the dough, add the brie, and fold the dough up the sides and over a portion of the brie.

4. Turn the brie over onto a pie plate or other rimmed baking dish so the cranberry side is facing upwards. Sprinkle the nuts and sweetener. **Must be fully enclosed in rind, *slices won't work.*

5. Bake for 25 min.

Chocolate Cake Donuts

Yields Provided: 8 Servings

Macro Counts For Each Serving:

- **Fat Content**: 9.2 g
- **Total Net Carbs**: 2.01 g
- **Protein**: 4.43 g
- **Calories**: 123

List of Ingredients - The Donuts:

- Coconut flour (.33 cup)
- Swerve sweetener (.33 cup)
- Cocoa powder (3 tbsp.)
- Bak. powder (1 tsp.)
- Salt (.25 tsp.)
- Large eggs (4)
- Melted butter (.25 cup)
- Vanilla extract (.25 tsp.)
- Brewed coffee or water (6 tbsp.)

List of Ingredients - The Glaze:

- Cocoa powder (1 tbsp.)
- Powdered swerve (.25 cup)
- Heavy cream (1 tbsp.)
- Vanilla extract (.25 tsp.)

- Water (1.5-2 tbsp.)

Preparation Technique:
1. Set the oven to 325° Fahrenheit. Spritz a donut pan with cooking oil spray.
2. Whisk the sweetener, coconut flour, salt, cocoa powder, and baking powder. Whisk and add in the eggs, melted butter, vanilla extract, and cold coffee/water.
3. Divide the batter among the wells of the donut pan.
4. Bake until the donuts are set (16-20 min.).
5. Transfer to the countertop. Cool in the pan for about ten minutes. Flip out onto a cooling rack.

Preparation Technique - The Glaze:
1. Whisk the powdered sweetener, cocoa powder, heavy cream, and vanilla.
2. Add just enough water to thin the glaze.
3. Dip the top of each donut into the glaze and let it sit for half an hour.

Cinnamon Donut Bites

Yields Provided: 12 Servings - 2 bites each

Macro Counts For Each Serving:

- **Fat Content**: 18 g
- **Total Net Carbs**: 3 g
- **Protein**: 7 g
- **Calories**: 164

List of Ingredients - The Bites:

- Swerve sweetener (.5 cup)
- Plain whey protein powder (.25 cup)
- Bak. powder (2 tsp.)
- Salt (.5 tsp.)
- Almond flour (2 cups)
- Cinnamon (.5 tsp.)
- Large eggs (2)
- Water (.33 cup)
- Butter - melted (.25 cup)
- Apple cider vinegar (1.5 tbsp.)
- Apple extract (1.5 tsp.)
- _Also Needed_: 24- count mini muffin pan

List of Ingredients - The Coating:

- Melted butter (.25 cup)

- Swerve sweetener (.25 cup)
- Cinnamon (1-2 tsp.)

Preparation Technique:

1. Warm the oven ahead of baking time to reach 325° Fahrenheit. Lightly grease the pan.
2. Whisk the almond flour, protein powder, baking powder, cinnamon, sweetener, and salt.
3. Whisk the eggs and water with the butter, apple cider vinegar, and apple extract. Combine the fixings.
4. Divide the mixture among the wells of the pan.
5. Bake until the muffins are firm to the touch (15-20 min.). Cool for ten minutes on a cooling rack.
6. In a small container, whisk the sweetener and cinnamon.
7. Dip each donut bite into the melted butter, coating completely.
8. Roll each donut bite into the cinnamon/sweetener mixture to serve.

Coconut Almond Crisps

Yields Provided: 12 Servings

Macro Counts For Each Serving:

- **Fat Content**: 6.12 g
- **Total Net Carbs**: 1.16 g
- **Protein**: 0.68 g
- **Calories**: 64

List of Ingredients:

- Butter (.25 cup)
- Swerve sweetener (.33 cup)
- Blackstrap molasses (2 tsp.)
- Xanthan gum (.25 tsp.)
- Almond meal (.25 cup)
- Shredded coconut (6 tbsp.)
- Vanilla extract (.5 tsp.)
- *Also Needed:* 2 baking tins with a layer of parchment paper

Preparation Technique:

1. Prepare the pans. Warm up the oven to 350° Fahrenheit.
2. Arrange the oven rack to the uppermost level in the oven.

3. Use medium heat on the stovetop in a saucepan to melt the butter, molasses, and swerve. When combined, remove from the burner and add the xanthan gum. Whisk and work in the shredded coconut, almond meal, and vanilla.
4. Use a teaspoon to drop the batter onto the prepared pans (4-in. between). Slightly, press down each one and bake for 8 to 12 minutes.
5. Once they are golden brown, remove from the oven.

Pancakes

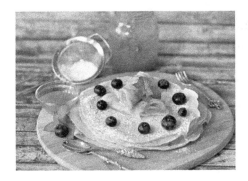

__Almond Cream Cheese Pancakes__

Yields Provided: 4 Servings (2 pancakes each)

Macro Counts For Each Serving:

- **Fat Content**: 15 g
- **Total Net Carbs**: 2.3 g
- **Protein**: 15.9 g
- **Calories**: 203

List of Ingredients:

- Almond flour (.5 cup + 1 tbsp.)
- Full-fat cream cheese (.5 cup)
- Eggs (4)
- Granulated sweetener (1 tsp.)
- Butter for frying (as needed)

Preparation Technique:

1. Mix all of the fixings in a blender.
2. Fry the pancakes in a pan with melted butter using the medium heat setting.
3. Flip once the center begins to bubble.
4. *Note:* Add .5 tsp. baking powder to make them super fluffy.

Blueberry Pancakes

Yields Provided: 2 pancakes - 1 serving

Macro Counts For Each Serving:

- **Fat Content**: 35 g
- **Total Net Carbs**: 7 g
- **Protein**: 15 g
- **Calories**: 415

List of Ingredients:

- Blueberries (30 g)
- Almond flour (.25 cup)
- Coconut flour (1 tsp.)
- Stevia (1/16 tsp. or to your liking)
- Cinnamon (.25 tsp.)
- Bak. powder (.25 tsp.)
- Salt (1 pinch)
- Coconut oil (1 tbsp.)
- Egg (1)
- Almond milk (1 tbsp.)

Preparation Technique:

1. Combine the dry fixings in the blender or Nutribullet.

2. Mix in the wet fixings and blend until combined. Fold in the berries.

3. Heat oil in a pan until hot and pour in half of the batter. Cook until bubbles begin to stay around the rim of the pancake (1.5 min.).

4. Flip and cook 30 seconds or until done. Prepare the second one and serve.

Coconut Pancakes

Yields Provided: 12 Servings (silver dollar sized)

Macro Counts For Each Serving:

- **Fat Content**: 7 g
- **Total Net Carbs**: 1 g
- **Protein**: 1 g
- **Calories**: 77

List of Ingredients:

- Unsalted Melted butter (.25 cup)
- Heavy cream or sour cream (.25 cup)
- Stevia (1 packet)
- Salt (.25 tsp.)
- Eggs (3 +1 if the batter is too thick)
- Coconut flour (.25 cup)
- Baking powder (.5 tsp.)
- Vanilla extract (.5 tsp.)
- Optional: Water

Preparation Technique:

1. Whisk the butter, eggs, salt, cream, stevia, and vanilla extract.

2. In a separate mixing container, sift the baking powder and flour.

3. Mix each of the dry fixings into the wet ones and let it rest to thicken (15-30 min.).

4. Warm a skillet using the medium heat setting. Add oil and the batter to form cakes 2-3 inches in diameter.

5. Flatten out the thick batter to form flatter rounds.

Conclusion

I hope you have thoroughly enjoyed each chapter of *Keto Bread*. I also hope it was informative and provided you with all of the tools you need to achieve your goals whatever they may be. The next step is to decide which delicious treat you want to make first. Head to the store for the fixings and you are ready to start.

If you are using the keto plan for weight loss, you may not see any results at first.
There could be days or weeks where you don't see the changes, but slow is the best method. You are altering your lifestyle and breaking old habits. You need to remain patient because there aren't any quick fixes to weight loss. As with any new challenge, the initial phase of a long-term trial is difficult.

You have to realize it takes time for your body to accommodate the ketogenic diet plan. It can take anywhere from two to four weeks or more. For some, it can take as much as six to eight weeks. It takes time because you cannot instantly switch over to using fat as a fuel source. It takes time for your body to adjust to the changes. You may be experiencing low energy, withdrawal-type symptoms, fatigue, or headaches, but they will pass.

Some recipes might not be 100% keto-friendly. You can also adjust the ingredients to your own discretion. Remember this Formula: Total Carbs minus (-) Fiber = Net Carbs. This is the logic used for each of the recipes included in this cookbook and guidelines.

Walk away with the knowledge learned and prepare a feast using your delicious new bread recipes and other delicious options. Be the envy of the neighborhood when you provide a feast at the next neighborhood gathering. Show off your skills and be proud. You can also boast of how much better you feel using the ketogenic diet plan.

After you have started losing your weight, it's essential to have a bit of fun. However, you should be sure it is not a food-related treat unless it's keto-friendly. Buy a new outfit to show off your weight loss. Take the family for an evening on-the-town. You deserve it.

Finally, if you found this book useful in any way, a review on Amazon is always appreciated!

CPSIA information can be obtained
at www.ICGtesting.com
Printed in the USA
BVHW040003190221
600507BV00012B/974

9 781801 650953